LOW OXALATE DIET FOR SENIOR OVER 50

A 21-Day Culinary Journey from Phase 1 to Flavorful Freedom

ANTHONY HILL

TABLE OF CONTENTS

INTRODUCTION

Meet Thomas, a passionate individual on a transformative health journey. Faced with the challenges of managing chronic inflammation, Thomas embarked on a quest to discover the power of an anti-inflammatory diet. This journey wasn't just about the latest health trend; it was about reclaiming control over his well-being and embracing a lifestyle that nurtured his body from within.

Thomas realized that meal preparation played a pivotal role in unlocking the potential of the anti-inflammatory diet. Inspired by the wealth of knowledge he gained, he embarked on a culinary adventure, transforming his kitchen into a haven of healing. The goal was simple yet profound: to curate meals that not only delighted the taste buds but also acted as a shield against inflammation.

His arsenal? Vibrant vegetables, antioxidant-rich fruits, lean proteins, and an array of anti-inflammatory herbs and spices. Thomas learned to harness the healing power of ingredients like turmeric, ginger, and leafy greens, creating a symphony of flavors that whispered promises of wellness.

As he immersed himself in the art of anti-inflammatory meal prep, Thomas discovered the beauty of balance.

Every meal became a masterpiece, a fusion of nutrient-dense elements carefully chosen to combat inflammation and promote overall health. His kitchen bore witness to the sizzle of sautéing colorful vegetables, the fragrance of herbs infusing into grains, and the vibrant hues of berries bursting with antioxidants.

But Thomas understood that the real magic lay in consistency. So, armed with colorful containers filled with his culinary creations, he embarked on a journey of mindful meal prep. Each Sunday, the kitchen transformed into a sanctuary of self-care, as Thomas prepared a week's worth of anti-inflammatory goodness, ready to fuel his body with the nutrition it deserved.

The benefits unfolded like chapters in a well-written novel. Thomas experienced increased energy levels, reduced joint pain, and a newfound sense of vitality. His story became an inspiration for others, as he shared not just recipes but the wisdom of how embracing an anti-inflammatory diet could be a delicious and empowering choice.

Thomas's journey was a testament to the transformative power of intentional eating. The anti-inflammatory diet meal prep wasn't just about food; it became a celebration of life, a daily ritual of nourishment, and a declaration of self-love. As he savored each bite of his meticulously prepared meals, Thomas found not just sustenance but a renewed sense of well-being – a taste of a life well-lived, free from the chains of inflammation.

Overview of Oxalates

Oxalates are naturally occurring compounds found in a wide variety of plant-based foods. These compounds are formed through the metabolism of plants, particularly those rich in oxalic acid. While oxalates play a role in the physiology of many plants, they can also have implications for human health, particularly in individuals prone to certain conditions.

- **Chemical Composition:** Oxalates belong to a group of organic acids known as oxalic acids. Chemically, they are composed of carbon, hydrogen, and oxygen atoms, with the molecular formula $C_2O_4^{2-}$.

- **Food Sources:** Oxalates are abundant in many foods, including fruits, vegetables, nuts, seeds, grains, and legumes. Some of the most common sources of dietary oxalates include spinach, rhubarb, beets, nuts, cocoa, and tea.

- **Formation and Function:** In plants, oxalates serve various functions, including defense against herbivores and pathogens, as well as regulating calcium levels. They are often found in the form of calcium oxalate crystals, which can act as a deterrent to predators.

- **Health Implications:** While oxalates are generally harmless for most people, they can pose health risks for individuals with certain conditions. High oxalate intake has been associated with the formation of kidney stones, particularly in those with a history of calcium oxalate stones. Additionally, some research suggests that oxalates may interfere with the absorption of minerals like calcium and magnesium.

- **Dietary Considerations:** For individuals susceptible to oxalate-related health issues, adopting a low oxalate diet may be recommended. This involves limiting the intake of high oxalate foods while incorporating alternative sources of nutrients into the diet.

- **Balancing Benefits and Risks:** While reducing oxalate intake may help mitigate certain health risks, it's important to strike a balance between avoiding high oxalate foods and maintaining a nutritious diet. Consulting with a healthcare professional or registered dietitian can provide personalized guidance on managing oxalate intake based on individual health needs.

Importance of Diet for Seniors

As we age, maintaining a healthy and well-balanced diet becomes increasingly vital for overall well-being and quality of life. The nutritional choices we make play a pivotal role in supporting various aspects of senior health, from physical and mental function to disease prevention. In the senior years, dietary considerations go beyond mere sustenance; they become a cornerstone for promoting longevity and optimizing the aging process. Here are key aspects highlighting the importance of diet for seniors:

- **Nutrient Absorption and Metabolism:**

Aging can affect the body's ability to absorb and metabolize nutrients efficiently. Adequate intake of essential vitamins, minerals, and other nutrients becomes crucial to compensate for potential deficiencies and support optimal bodily functions.

- **Maintaining Healthy Weight:**

Seniors often face challenges related to weight management, including changes in metabolism and decreased physical activity. A balanced diet helps in maintaining a healthy weight, preventing obesity-related conditions, and supporting overall mobility.

- **Bone Health and Osteoporosis Prevention:**

Calcium and vitamin D are essential for maintaining bone health, and seniors are particularly susceptible to conditions like osteoporosis. A diet rich in these nutrients, along with other bone-supporting minerals, contributes to bone density and reduces the risk of fractures.

- **Heart Health and Blood Pressure Management:**

Heart health becomes a paramount concern as we age. A diet low in saturated fats, cholesterol, and sodium, and high in fiber, antioxidants, and omega-3 fatty acids, can help manage blood pressure, lower cholesterol levels, and reduce the risk of cardiovascular diseases.

- **Cognitive Function and Brain Health:**

Certain nutrients, such as omega-3 fatty acids, antioxidants, and vitamins like B12, are associated with cognitive function and brain health. A well-balanced diet can contribute to maintaining mental acuity and reducing the risk of age-related cognitive decline.

- **Immune System Support:**

A healthy diet strengthens the immune system, which is particularly important for seniors as they may be more vulnerable to infections and illnesses. Nutrient-rich foods provide the necessary vitamins and minerals to support immune function.

- **Digestive Health:**

Seniors often experience changes in digestive function, including a slower metabolism and potential issues like constipation. A diet high in fiber, fluids, and probiotics supports digestive health and regular bowel movements.

- **Chronic Disease Prevention and Management:**

Proper nutrition plays a crucial role in preventing and managing chronic conditions such as diabetes, arthritis, and certain cancers. A well-designed diet can help control blood sugar levels, reduce inflammation, and support overall health.

- **Hydration and Kidney Health:**

Adequate hydration is essential for kidney health, especially as the aging process can impact the body's ability to conserve water. Seniors should maintain proper fluid intake to support kidney function and prevent dehydration.

- **Emotional Well-being:**

Diet can also influence mood and emotional well-being. Nutrient-rich foods contribute to the production of neurotransmitters that regulate mood, helping seniors maintain a positive mental outlook.

Purpose of the Low Oxalate Diet

A low oxalate diet serves as a specialized approach to nutrition, aiming to manage and reduce the intake of oxalates in the diet. For individuals, particularly seniors at the age of 50 and beyond, adopting a low oxalate diet may have various purposes and potential benefits. Here are key reasons behind the purpose of the low oxalate diet:

- **Kidney Stone Prevention:**

One of the primary motivations for adopting a low oxalate diet is the prevention of kidney stones. Oxalates can bind with calcium to form crystals, and in individuals prone to kidney stones, these crystals may accumulate, leading to the formation of stones. By reducing dietary oxalate intake, the risk of forming calcium oxalate stones in the kidneys is mitigated.

- **Minimizing Oxalate-Related Health Issues:**

Some individuals may be more sensitive to oxalates, experiencing symptoms or complications related to their consumption. Conditions such as Hyperxaluria, where there is an excessive excretion of oxalates in the urine, or certain kidney disorders may necessitate a low oxalate diet to manage symptoms and prevent complications.

- **Supporting Joint Health:**

Oxalates have been associated with joint pain and inflammation, and for seniors managing conditions like osteoarthritis or rheumatoid arthritis, adopting a low oxalate diet may contribute to reducing discomfort and supporting overall joint health.

- **Improving Nutrient Absorption:**

High oxalate intake may interfere with the absorption of certain minerals, such as calcium and magnesium. By reducing oxalate levels in the diet, seniors can enhance the absorption of these essential nutrients, supporting bone health and overall well-being.

- **Individualized Health Plans:**

The low oxalate diet allows for a personalized and targeted approach to nutrition. Seniors with specific health concerns, such as kidney issues or a history of kidney stones, can work with healthcare professionals and dietitians to tailor their dietary choices to better align with their individual health needs.

- **Managing Chronic Conditions:**

Individuals with certain chronic conditions, such as autoimmune disorders or digestive issues, may find that a low oxalate diet helps manage symptoms and supports their overall health. This is particularly relevant for seniors dealing with multiple health considerations.

- **Promoting Overall Wellness:**

Beyond specific health concerns, adopting a low oxalate diet can contribute to an overall sense of wellness. By paying attention to dietary choices and opting for nutrient-dense, low oxalate foods, seniors can actively participate in their health and well-being.

- **Reducing Oxalate-Related Pain and Discomfort:**

For some individuals, high oxalate intake has been linked to pain and discomfort, particularly in sensitive areas such as the urinary tract or joints. A low oxalate diet may help alleviate these symptoms and improve the overall quality of life for seniors.

CHAPTER ONE

UNDERSTANDING OXALATES

What are Oxalates?

Oxalates are naturally occurring compounds found in a wide range of plant-based foods. Chemically, they are the salts or esters of oxalic acid, a substance present in many vegetables, fruits, nuts, seeds, grains, and legumes. Oxalates are produced by plants as part of their defense mechanism against herbivores and pathogens, and they are also involved in the regulation of calcium within the plant's tissues.

In the human body, oxalates can bind with minerals, particularly calcium, to form insoluble crystals. While most of these crystals are excreted through urine or bile without causing harm, high levels of oxalates in the body can lead to the formation of crystals that contribute to the development of kidney stones. The most common type of kidney stone is calcium oxalate, formed when calcium binds with oxalate in the urine.

While kidney stones are one of the most well-known consequences of high oxalate intake, some individuals may also experience other health issues related to oxalates. These may include gastrointestinal symptoms, such as bloating or diarrhea, as well as joint pain or inflammation, especially in those with pre-existing conditions like osteoarthritis or rheumatoid arthritis.

It's important to note that oxalates themselves are not inherently harmful, and many foods containing oxalates also provide essential nutrients and health benefits. However, for individuals prone to kidney stones or sensitive to oxalate-related symptoms, managing oxalate intake through dietary modifications, such as a low oxalate diet, may be recommended.

Sources of Oxalates in Food

Oxalates are present in a variety of plant-based foods, and their concentration can vary widely among different food items. Here is a list of common sources of oxalates in food:

Leafy Greens:

- Spinach
- Swiss chard
- Beet greens
- Collard greens
- Kale

- Turnip greens
- ***Vegetables:***
- Beets
- Okra
- Sweet potatoes
- Potatoes (especially if the skin is consumed)
- Rhubarb

Fruits:

- Berries (strawberries, blueberries, raspberries)
- Grapes
- Figs
- Oranges and orange juice
- Kiwi
- Bananas

Nuts and Seeds:

- Almonds
- Cashews
- Peanuts
- Sesame seeds
- Sunflower seeds

Grains and Cereals:

- Whole wheat

- Brown rice
- Quinoa
- Buckwheat

Legumes:

- Soybeans
- Black beans
- Navy beans
- Lentils

Beverages:

- Tea (black and green)
- Coffee (particularly instant coffee)

Other Foods:

- Cocoa and chocolate
- Tofu
- Nutritional yeast

How Oxalates Affect the Body

Oxalates can affect the body in various ways, both positively and negatively. While they are naturally occurring compounds found in many plant-based foods and have some health benefits, excessive levels of oxalates can lead to health issues. Here's an overview of how oxalates can affect the body:

Positive Aspects:

- **Antioxidant Properties:**

Some foods rich in oxalates, such as certain fruits and vegetables, also contain antioxidants. Antioxidants help neutralize free radicals in the body, protecting cells from damage and contributing to overall health.

- **Plant Defense Mechanism:**

In plants, oxalates serve as a defense mechanism against herbivores and pathogens. The formation of calcium oxalate crystals can act as a deterrent to grazing animals and help protect the plant.

- **Calcium Regulation in Plants:**

Oxalates play a role in regulating calcium within plant tissues. This helps maintain the structural integrity of plant cells and contributes to the plant's overall health.

Negative Aspects:

- **Kidney Stone Formation:**

The most well-known negative effect of oxalates is their association with kidney stones. When oxalates bind with calcium in the urine, they can form insoluble crystals, contributing to the development of calcium oxalate kidney stones. Individuals prone to kidney stones or with a history of kidney stone formation may need to manage their oxalate intake.

- **Reduced Mineral Absorption:**

Oxalates can bind with minerals like calcium and form insoluble complexes, reducing the absorption of these minerals in the digestive tract. This can potentially lead to issues related to calcium deficiency, impacting bone health and other bodily functions.

- **Gastrointestinal Symptoms:**

Some individuals may be sensitive to high levels of dietary oxalates, experiencing gastrointestinal symptoms such as bloating, gas, or diarrhea. This is more common in individuals with certain digestive disorders.

- **Joint Pain and Inflammation:**

Oxalates have been linked to joint pain and inflammation, particularly in individuals with pre-existing conditions such as osteoarthritis or rheumatoid arthritis. Reducing oxalate intake may help alleviate these symptoms in some cases.

- **Interference with Nutrient Absorption:**

In addition to calcium, oxalates can interfere with the absorption of other minerals, such as magnesium. This interference may impact overall nutrient absorption and utilization in the body.

Oxalate-Related Health Concerns for Seniors

Seniors, particularly those at the age of 50 and beyond, may face specific health concerns related to oxalates. Understanding these concerns is crucial for adopting a dietary approach that supports overall well-being. Here are some oxalate-related health concerns for seniors:

- **Kidney Stone Formation:**

Seniors are at an increased risk of developing kidney stones due to age-related changes in kidney function. Oxalates can contribute to the formation of calcium oxalate crystals, a common type of kidney stone. Seniors with a history of kidney stones or those predisposed to stone formation should be mindful of their oxalate intake.

- **Reduced Calcium Absorption:**

Calcium is essential for maintaining bone health, and seniors are already at risk for bone-related issues such as osteoporosis. High oxalate levels in the diet can bind with calcium, leading to reduced absorption. This may exacerbate calcium deficiency concerns in seniors, impacting bone strength.

- **Joint Pain and Inflammation:**

Oxalates have been associated with joint pain and inflammation. Seniors, especially those with arthritis or joint-related conditions, may experience discomfort that could be influenced by their oxalate intake. Managing oxalates may be a consideration in alleviating joint symptoms.

- **Digestive Issues:**

Some seniors may experience digestive issues related to high oxalate intake, including bloating, gas, or diarrhea. Individuals with pre-existing digestive conditions may be more sensitive to oxalates, and adjusting their diet could help manage these symptoms.

- **Potential Nutrient Deficiencies:**

Oxalates can bind with minerals like calcium and interfere with their absorption in the digestive tract. Seniors already face challenges related to nutrient absorption, and high oxalate intake may exacerbate these issues, potentially leading to nutrient deficiencies.

- **Implications for Bone Health:**

Seniors are particularly vulnerable to bone-related concerns, and oxalates can influence mineral balance, impacting bone health. Ensuring an adequate intake of nutrients like calcium and magnesium, while managing oxalate intake, becomes crucial for maintaining bone density.

- **Impact on Kidney Function:**

Seniors may experience age-related changes in kidney function, making it important to monitor oxalate intake. High oxalate levels can potentially strain the kidneys, and individuals with kidney issues may need to manage oxalates to support kidney health.

- **Individual Sensitivities:**

Each senior's response to oxalates can vary. Some may be more sensitive to the impact of oxalates on their health, while others may tolerate higher levels without adverse effects. Recognizing individual sensitivities and adjusting the diet accordingly is essential.

CHAPTER TWO

THE BENEFITS OF A LOW OXALATE DIET

Improved Kidney Health

Adopting a low oxalate diet can contribute to improved kidney health, particularly for individuals who are prone to kidney stones or have kidney-related concerns. Here's how a low oxalate diet can positively impact kidney health:

- **Reduced Risk of Kidney Stone Formation:**

The primary benefit of a low oxalate diet for kidney health is the decreased risk of kidney stone formation. Oxalates can bind with calcium in the urine to form insoluble crystals, contributing to the development of kidney stones. By limiting dietary oxalates, the likelihood of these crystals forming is reduced, lowering the risk of kidney stone recurrence.

- **Prevention of Calcium Oxalate Stones:**

The most common type of kidney stone is the calcium oxalate stone. By managing oxalate intake, particularly for individuals with a history of calcium oxalate stones, a low oxalate diet can help prevent the formation of these stones and promote kidney health.

- **Support for Individuals with Hyperxaluria:**

Hyperoxaluria is a condition characterized by elevated levels of oxalates in the urine, increasing the risk of kidney stone formation. For individuals with Hyperxaluria, adopting a low oxalate diet, along with medical supervision, may be recommended to manage oxalate excretion and support kidney function.

- **Potential Reduction in Kidney Strain:**

High oxalate levels in the diet may potentially strain the kidneys, especially in individuals with compromised kidney function. A low oxalate diet can help alleviate this strain and contribute to overall kidney function.

- **Minimized Crystal Formation:**

Oxalates in the urine can form crystals even in individuals who haven't experienced kidney stones. These crystals may contribute to kidney damage over time. By reducing dietary oxalates, the formation of these crystals is minimized, supporting kidney health.

Maintenance of Optimal Hydration:

Staying well-hydrated is essential for kidney health, as it helps flush toxins and waste products from the body. A low oxalate diet often emphasizes the importance of adequate hydration, which is beneficial for overall kidney function.

- **Individualized Approach for Seniors:**

Seniors, who may already be more vulnerable to kidney-related issues due to age-related changes, can benefit from an individualized approach to nutrition. A low oxalate diet can be tailored to their specific health needs, taking into account factors such as kidney function and any history of kidney stones.

Joint and Bone Health

A low oxalate diet can contribute to improved joint and bone health, especially for seniors who may be more susceptible to conditions such as osteoarthritis or osteoporosis. Here's how a low oxalate diet can positively impact joint and bone health:

- **Reduced Inflammation:**

Oxalates have been associated with joint pain and inflammation. By managing oxalate intake, particularly from high-oxalate foods, individuals may experience a reduction in inflammation, contributing to improved joint comfort and mobility.

- **Alleviation of Arthritic Symptoms:**

Seniors with arthritis, whether osteoarthritis or rheumatoid arthritis, may find that a low oxalate diet helps alleviate joint pain and stiffness. While individual responses vary, some individuals report improved joint function and reduced arthritic symptoms when adopting a low oxalate approach.

- **Calcium Absorption for Bone Density:**

Calcium is crucial for maintaining bone density and preventing conditions like osteoporosis. Oxalates can bind with calcium, potentially reducing its absorption in the digestive tract. By managing oxalate intake, seniors can enhance calcium absorption and support bone health.

- **Minimized Impact on Bone Mineralization:**

Excessive oxalates in the body can interfere with the mineralization process essential for bone strength. By adopting a low oxalate diet, seniors can help minimize the impact of oxalates on bone mineralization, reducing the risk of bone-related issues.

- **Prevention of Calcium Oxalate Crystals in Joints:**

In addition to kidney stones, calcium oxalate crystals can potentially form in joints, contributing to joint pain and inflammation. By managing oxalate intake, seniors can help prevent the formation of these crystals, promoting joint health.

- **Nutrient-Rich Alternatives:**

A low oxalate diet encourages the inclusion of nutrient-rich alternatives that benefit joint and bone health. Foods such as low-oxalate leafy greens, dairy products, and fortified foods can provide essential nutrients like calcium, vitamin D, and magnesium that support bone strength and overall musculoskeletal function.

- **Personalized Approach for Seniors:**

Seniors may have unique considerations related to joint and bone health. A low oxalate diet can be tailored to their individual needs, taking into account factors such as existing health conditions, medication use, and nutritional requirements.

- **Holistic Approach to Wellness:**

Adopting a low oxalate diet is part of a holistic approach to wellness. By making conscious dietary choices, seniors can actively contribute to their overall health, supporting not only joint and bone health but also other aspects of well-being.

Digestive Wellness

A low oxalate diet can contribute to digestive wellness by addressing potential concerns related to high oxalate intake. Here's how adopting a low oxalate diet can positively impact digestive health:

- **Reduced Risk of Gastrointestinal Symptoms:**

Some individuals may be sensitive to high levels of dietary oxalates, experiencing symptoms such as bloating, gas, or diarrhea. By adopting a low oxalate diet, individuals can minimize the risk of gastrointestinal discomfort and promote digestive comfort.

- **Alleviation of Irritable Bowel Symptoms:**

Individuals with irritable bowel syndrome (IBS) or other digestive disorders may find that a low oxalate diet helps alleviate symptoms. High oxalate intake can potentially contribute to digestive distress, and managing oxalates may be part of a comprehensive approach to managing IBS symptoms.

- **Improved Nutrient Absorption:**

Oxalates can bind with minerals, such as calcium and magnesium, in the digestive tract, potentially reducing their absorption. By adopting a low oxalate diet, individuals can enhance nutrient absorption, supporting overall nutritional status and digestive wellness.

- **Prevention of Oxalate Crystal Formation:**

Oxalates in the digestive system can potentially form crystals, which may contribute to kidney stones or other health issues. By managing oxalate intake, individuals can help prevent the formation of these crystals, supporting both digestive and kidney health.

- **Balanced Microbiota:**

Some high-oxalate foods may interact with gut bacteria, influencing the balance of the microbiota. Adopting a low oxalate diet may contribute to a more balanced and diverse gut microbiome, which is essential for digestive health and overall well-being.

- **Individualized Approach for Seniors:**

Seniors may face age-related changes in digestive function, and a low oxalate diet can be tailored to their specific needs. Managing oxalate intake may help seniors maintain digestive comfort and support optimal nutrient absorption.

- **Enhanced Hydration:**

A low oxalate diet often emphasizes the importance of staying well-hydrated. Proper hydration is essential for maintaining digestive regularity and preventing issues such as constipation, which can be more prevalent in seniors.

- **Promotion of Overall Wellness:**

Digestive wellness is integral to overall health, and adopting a low oxalate diet can be part of a comprehensive approach to promoting well-being. Making mindful dietary choices supports digestive comfort and contributes to an improved quality of life.

Managing Chronic Conditions

A low oxalate diet can be a valuable component in managing certain chronic conditions, especially those related to kidney health, joint function, and digestive well-

- **Kidney Stone Prevention:**

Individuals with a history of kidney stones, particularly calcium oxalate stones, can benefit from a low oxalate diet. By reducing dietary oxalates, the risk of forming kidney stones is minimized, contributing to the management of this chronic condition.

- **Support for Hyperoxaluria:**

Hyperoxaluria, characterized by elevated levels of oxalates in the urine, can increase the risk of kidney stone formation. Managing oxalate intake through a low oxalate diet, in conjunction with medical guidance, can help support individuals with Hyperxaluria.

- **Joint Pain and Inflammation:**

Chronic conditions affecting the joints, such as osteoarthritis or rheumatoid arthritis, may be influenced by inflammation. Some individuals with these conditions report relief from joint pain and inflammation when following a low oxalate diet, contributing to the overall management of their condition.

- **Digestive Disorders:**

Individuals with irritable bowel syndrome (IBS) or other digestive disorders may find that managing oxalate intake helps alleviate symptoms. For those with specific digestive concerns related to oxalates, a low oxalate diet can be part of a comprehensive approach to managing their chronic digestive condition.

- **Balanced Nutrient Absorption:**

Chronic conditions often coincide with concerns related to nutrient absorption. Oxalates can bind with minerals, potentially reducing their absorption. A low oxalate diet can help optimize nutrient absorption, supporting individuals managing chronic health conditions.

- **Customized Approach for Seniors:**

Seniors with chronic conditions may benefit from a customized approach to nutrition. A low oxalate diet, tailored to individual health needs, can be part of a comprehensive strategy for managing chronic conditions in the aging population.

- **Improved Quality of Life:**

Managing chronic conditions involves various aspects of lifestyle, including dietary choices. Adopting a low oxalate diet, where appropriate, can contribute to an improved quality of life by addressing specific aspects related to kidney health, joint function, and digestive comfort.

- **Holistic Health Approach:**

A low oxalate diet fits into a holistic approach to health that considers the interconnectedness of different bodily systems. By managing oxalate intake, individuals can actively participate in their overall well-being and support the management of chronic conditions.

CHAPTER THREE

LOW OXALATE DIET AND PREPARATION

In the heart of a charming neighborhood, George, a spirited retiree with a zest for life, found himself at a crossroads. Having recently faced health challenges related to kidney stones, he was determined to take charge of his well-being. Little did he know that a journey into the world of low oxalate diet meal prep would not only transform his health but also ignite a culinary revolution in his community.

George's love for delicious meals and social gatherings was undeniable, and he refused to let health setbacks dim his passion. One day, as he delved into research, George stumbled upon the concept of a low oxalate diet. Intrigued, he envisioned a world where flavorful, health-conscious meals could be at the center of his life.

Armed with newfound knowledge, George began experimenting in his kitchen, crafting low oxalate meals that were as delightful to the taste buds as they were nourishing to his body. The aroma of fresh herbs, vibrant vegetables, and lean proteins filled his home, creating a sanctuary of wellness and culinary creativity.

As George's culinary skills blossomed, he couldn't keep the magic to himself. His friends and neighbors took notice of his vibrant energy and newfound enthusiasm. Intrigued, they gathered in his kitchen, eager to learn the secrets of this transformative low oxalate meal prep.

Under George's guidance, the kitchen became a hub of laughter, discovery, and friendship. Together, they chopped, sautéed, and shared stories of their health journeys. George's low oxalate meal prep sessions became a weekly ritual, a celebration of good food, great company, and the shared commitment to vibrant health.

Word of George's culinary prowess spread, and soon the entire neighborhood was buzzing with excitement. Local gatherings turned into low oxalate potlucks, and the community flourished with a renewed sense of vitality and well-being.

Inspired by the positive impact on his own life and those around him, George decided to spread the joy further. He started organizing workshops, sharing his knowledge with other retirees in neighboring communities. The simple act of preparing meals became a catalyst for profound change, transforming lives one delicious bite at a time.

As George stood among his neighbors, pots simmering and laughter echoing, he marveled at the power of a low oxalate diet to bring people together and enhance their quality of life. His journey had not only rejuvenated his health but had created a ripple effect of wellness, connecting a community through the joy of mindful, delicious eating.

CHAPTER FOUR

BREAKFAST RECIPES

Blueberry Jam Parfait

Ingredients:

- 4 cups fresh blueberries
- 1 1/2 cups sugar
- 1/4 cup lemon juice
- 1 packet pectin

Preparation Time: 15 minutes

Cooking Time: 20 minutes

Serving Time: 8 hours (overnight refrigeration)

Nutritional Info: (per serving) Calories: 150, Carbohydrates: 38g, Sugars: 32g

Instructions:

- In a large pot, combine blueberries, sugar, and lemon juice.
- Bring to a boil, stirring occasionally. Add pectin and boil for an additional 5 minutes.
- Pour into sterilized jars and seal. Allow to cool before refrigerating overnight.

Serving Methods:

1. Serve as a parfait with layers of Greek yogurt and granola.

2. Spread on whole-grain toast for a quick and tasty breakfast.

Peach Mango Chia Seed Jam

Ingredients:

- 2 cups peaches, peeled and diced
- 1 cup mango, peeled and diced
- 1/2 cup honey
- 2 tablespoons chia seeds

Preparation Time: 20 minutes

Cooking Time: 25 minutes

Serving Time: 6 hours (setting time)

Nutritional Info: (per serving) Calories: 80, Protein: 1g, Fiber: 3g

Instructions:

- In a saucepan, combine peaches, mango, and honey. Simmer until fruit is soft.
- Mash the mixture and stir in chia seeds. Cook for an additional 5 minutes.
- Pour into jars and refrigerate until set.

1. Top overnight oats with a spoonful of jam.
2. Mix with Greek yogurt for a fruity chia pudding.

Cinnamon Apple Butter

Ingredients:

- 6 cups apples, peeled and chopped
- 1 cup apple cider
- 1 cup brown sugar
- 2 teaspoons cinnamon

Preparation Time: 15 minutes

Cooking Time: 2 hours

Serving Time: 4 hours (cooling time)

Nutritional Info: (per serving) Calories: 120, Fat: 0.5g, Vitamin C: 4%

Instructions:

- Combine apples, apple cider, brown sugar, and cinnamon in a slow cooker.
- Cook on low for 8 hours, stirring occasionally.
- Blend the mixture until smooth and cool before canning.

Serving Methods:

1. Spread on whole-grain English muffins.

2. Use as a topping for pancakes or waffles.

Strawberry Basil Preserves

Ingredients:

- 5 cups strawberries, hulled and halved

- 1 1/2 cups sugar

- 1/4 cup fresh basil, chopped

- 1 tablespoon lemon juice

Preparation Time: 20 minutes

Cooking Time: 15 minutes

Serving Time: 3 hours (cooling time)

Nutritional Info: (per serving) Calories: 70, Carbohydrates: 18g, Protein: 0.5g

Instructions:

- In a pot, combine strawberries, sugar, basil, and lemon juice.

- Bring to a boil and simmer until strawberries break down.

- Allow the mixture to cool before jarring.

Serving Methods:

1. Mix into plain yogurt for a fruity twist.

2. Spread on a warm croissant for a delightful breakfast treat.

Apricot Almond Butter

Ingredients:

- 4 cups apricots, pitted and chopped
- 1/2 cup almonds, chopped
- 1 cup honey
- 1 teaspoon almond extract

Preparation Time: 25 minutes

Cooking Time: 20 minutes

Serving Time: 5 hours (cooling time)

Nutritional Info: (per serving) Calories: 100, Protein: 2g, Fiber: 1.5g

Instructions:

- Cook apricots, almonds, honey, and almond extract until soft.
- Blend until smooth and let cool before canning.

Serving Methods:

1. Spread on whole-grain bagels.
2. Dip apple slices for a nutritious morning snack.

Raspberry Lemon Marmalade

Ingredients:

- 3 cups raspberries
- 2 cups sugar
- Zest and juice of 2 lemons

Preparation Time: 15 minutes

Cooking Time: 25 minutes

Serving Time: 4 hours (setting time)

Nutritional Info: (per serving) Calories: 90, Carbohydrates: 23g, Vitamin C: 30%

Instructions:

- Combine raspberries, sugar, lemon zest, and lemon juice in a saucepan.
- Bring to a boil, then simmer until it reaches a marmalade consistency.
- Allow the mixture to set in jars before refrigerating.

Serving Methods:

1. Spread on toast for a zesty start to the day.
2. Mix with cream cheese and spread on a warm baguette.

Cherry Vanilla Compote

Ingredients:

- 4 cups cherries, pitted and halved
- 1 cup sugar
- 1 vanilla bean, split
- 1/4 cup water

Preparation Time: 20 minutes

Cooking Time: 20 minutes

Serving Time: 3 hours (cooling time)

Nutritional Info: (per serving) Calories: 110, Carbohydrates: 27g, Fiber: 2g

Instructions:

- Combine cherries, sugar, vanilla bean, and water in a saucepan.
- Simmer until cherries are tender and the mixture thickens.
- Remove the vanilla bean and let the compote cool before canning.

Serving Methods:

1. Spoon over Greek yogurt for a decadent breakfast.
2. Top vanilla ice cream for a sweet treat.

Pumpkin Spice Jam

Ingredients:

- 3 cups pumpkin puree
- 1 1/2 cups brown sugar
- 1 teaspoon cinnamon
- 1/2 teaspoon nutmeg

Preparation Time: 15 minutes

Cooking Time: 20 minutes

Serving Time: 4 hours (cooling time)

Nutritional Info: (per serving) Calories: 70, Carbohydrates: 18g, Vitamin A: 200%

Instructions:

- Cook pumpkin puree, brown sugar, cinnamon, and nutmeg until thick.
- Allow the mixture to cool before canning.

Serving Methods:

1. Spread on warm toast for a fall-inspired breakfast.
2. Swirl into oatmeal for a hearty morning meal.

Mango Pineapple Jam

Ingredients:

- 3 cups mango, peeled and diced
- 2 cups pineapple, diced
- 1 1/2 cups sugar
- 1/4 cup lime juice

Preparation Time: 20 minutes

Cooking Time: 25 minutes

Serving Time: 6 hours (setting time)

Nutritional Info: (per serving)

Calories: 100, Vitamin C: 40%, Fiber: 1.5g

Instructions:

- Cook mango, pineapple, sugar, and lime juice until the mixture thickens.
- Allow the jam to set in jars before refrigerating.

Serving Methods:

1. Spread on whole-grain English muffins.
2. Use as a topping for yogurt parfait.

Fig Walnut Preserves

Ingredients:

- 4 cups fresh figs, chopped
- 1 cup walnuts, chopped

- 1 1/2 cups honey
- 1/4 cup balsamic vinegar

Preparation Time: 20 minutes

Cooking Time: 30 minutes

Serving Time: 5 hours (cooling time)

Nutritional Info: (per serving) Calories: 120, Protein: 2.5g, Fiber: 3g

Instructions:

- Combine figs, walnuts, honey, and balsamic vinegar in a saucepan.
- Cook until figs are soft and the mixture thickens.
- Let the preserves cool before canning.

Serving Methods:

1. Spread on a warm baguette with goat cheese.
2. Mix into plain yogurt for a delightful morning treat.

CHAPTER FIVE

LUNCH RECIPES

Roasted Red Pepper and Tomato Soup

Ingredients:

- 4 large red bell peppers, roasted and peeled
- 2 cans (28 oz. each) diced tomatoes
- 1 onion, chopped
- 2 cloves garlic, minced
- 4 cups low-sodium vegetable broth
- 1 teaspoon dried oregano
- Salt and pepper to taste

Preparation Time: 15 minutes

Cooking Time: 30 minutes

Serving Time: 45 minutes

Nutritional Info: (Per serving) Calories: 120, Protein: 3g, Fat: 2g, Carbs: 25g

Instructions:

- In a large pot, sauté onions and garlic until softened.
- Add roasted red peppers, diced tomatoes, vegetable broth, oregano, salt, and pepper.

- Simmer for 20-25 minutes.

- Blend until smooth using an immersion blender.

- Serve hot.

Serving Methods:

1. Garnish with a dollop of low-fat Greek yogurt.

2. Sprinkle with fresh basil leaves.

Chicken and Vegetable Stew

Ingredients:

- 1 lb. boneless, skinless chicken breast, cubed

- 2 cups carrots, sliced

- 2 cups green beans, chopped

- 1 cup celery, diced

- 1 onion, finely chopped

- 4 cups low-sodium chicken broth

- 2 tablespoons olive oil

- 1 teaspoon thyme

- Salt and pepper to taste

Preparation Time: 20 minutes

Cooking Time: 40 minutes

Serving Time: 60 minutes

Nutritional Info: (Per serving) Calories: 250, Protein: 25g, Fat: 8g, Carbs: 20g

Instructions:

- In a large pot, sauté chicken in olive oil until browned.
- Add onions, carrots, green beans, and celery. Cook until vegetables are tender.
- Pour in chicken broth, thyme, salt, and pepper. Simmer for 30 minutes.
- Serve hot.

Serving Methods:

1. Pair with a side of steamed quinoa.
2. Garnish with chopped parsley.

Zucchini and Tomato Salad

Ingredients:

- 4 medium zucchinis, sliced
- 2 cups cherry tomatoes, halved
- 1/4 cup feta cheese, crumbled
- 2 tablespoons olive oil
- 2 tablespoons balsamic vinegar
- 1 teaspoon dried basil
- Salt and pepper to taste

Preparation Time: 15 minutes

Cooking Time: 0 minutes

Serving Time: 15 minutes

Nutritional Info: (Per serving) Calories: 120, Protein: 5g, Fat: 8g, Carbs: 10g

Instructions:

- In a large bowl, combine zucchini and cherry tomatoes.
- In a small bowl, whisk together olive oil, balsamic vinegar, dried basil, salt, and pepper.
- Pour the dressing over the vegetables, toss gently.
- Sprinkle with feta cheese before serving.

Serving Methods:

1. Serve as a side dish with grilled chicken.
2. Mix in cooked quinoa for a heartier option.

Salmon and Asparagus Foil Packets

Ingredients:

- 4 salmon fillets
- 2 bunches asparagus, trimmed
- 2 tablespoons olive oil
- 2 cloves garlic, minced

- 1 lemon, sliced
- Fresh dill for garnish
- Salt and pepper to taste

Preparation Time: 15 minutes

Cooking Time: 20 minutes

Serving Time: 35 minutes

Nutritional Info: (Per serving) Calories: 300, Protein: 30g, Fat: 15g, Carbs: 10g

Instructions:

- Preheat the oven to 400°F (200°C).
- Place each salmon fillet on a piece of foil, surrounded by asparagus.
- Drizzle olive oil over salmon and asparagus, add minced garlic, salt, and pepper.
- Top with lemon slices and fold the foil to create packets.
- Bake for 15-20 minutes until salmon is cooked through.
- Garnish with fresh dill before serving.

Serving Methods:

1. Serve over a bed of cauliflower rice for a low-carb option.

2. Accompany with a side of mixed greens drizzled with vinaigrette.

Cauliflower and Broccoli Soup

Ingredients:

- 1 head cauliflower, chopped
- 2 cups broccoli florets
- 1 onion, chopped
- 2 cloves garlic, minced
- 4 cups low-sodium vegetable broth
- 1 cup unsweetened almond milk
- 2 tablespoons olive oil
- 1 teaspoon thyme
- Salt and pepper to taste

Preparation Time: 20 minutes2

Cooking Time: 25 minutes

Serving Time: 45 minutes

Nutritional Info: (Per serving) Calories: 150, Protein: 5g, Fat: 8g, Carbs: 15g

Instructions:

- In a large pot, sauté onions and garlic in olive oil until softened.

- Add cauliflower, broccoli, vegetable broth, almond milk, thyme, salt, and pepper.
- Simmer until vegetables are tender, about 20 minutes.
- Blend the soup until smooth using an immersion blender.
- Serve hot.

Serving Methods:

1. Top with a dollop of Greek yogurt.
2. Sprinkle with chopped chives for added freshness.

Eggplant and Bell Pepper Relish

Ingredients:

- 2 medium eggplants, diced
- 2 bell peppers (any color), diced
- 1 onion, finely chopped
- 2 cloves garlic, minced
- 1 cup white wine vinegar
- 1/4 cup honey
- 1 teaspoon cumin
- Salt and pepper to taste

Preparation Time: 20 minutes

Cooking Time: 30 minutes

Serving Time: 50 minutes

Nutritional Info: (Per serving) Calories: 80, Protein: 2g, Fat: 1g, Carbs: 18g

Instructions:

- In a large saucepan, combine eggplants, bell peppers, onions, and garlic.
- Add vinegar, honey, cumin, salt, and pepper. Bring to a boil.
- Reduce heat and simmer until vegetables are tender and the mixture thickens.
- Allow to cool before transferring to jars for canning.

Serving Methods:

1. Serve as a relish on top of grilled chicken.
2. Mix into quinoa or couscous for a flavorful side dish.

Turkey and Vegetable Lettuce Wraps

Ingredients:

- 1 lb. ground turkey
- 1 cup zucchini, diced
- 1 cup bell peppers (any color), diced
- 1 cup cherry tomatoes, quartered

- 1/2 cup low-sodium soy sauce
- 2 tablespoons sesame oil
- 2 teaspoons ginger, minced
- Butter lettuce leaves for wrapping

Preparation Time: 15 minutes

Cooking Time: 20 minutes

Serving Time: 35 minutes

Nutritional Info: (Per serving, 2 wraps) Calories: 180, Protein: 15g, Fat: 10g, Carbs: 8g

Instructions:

- In a skillet, cook ground turkey until browned.
- Add zucchini, bell peppers, cherry tomatoes, soy sauce, sesame oil, and ginger. Stir until vegetables are tender.
- Spoon the mixture into butter lettuce leaves.
- Serve immediately.

Serving Methods:

1. Top with chopped green onions for extra freshness.
2. Drizzle with a low-oxalate hoisin sauce for added flavor.

Spaghetti Squash with Pesto and Cherry Tomatoes

Ingredients:

- 1 medium spaghetti squash, halved and seeds removed
- 1 cup cherry tomatoes, halved
- 1/2 cup homemade low-oxalate pesto
- 2 tablespoons olive oil
- Salt and pepper to taste
- Fresh basil for garnish

Preparation Time: 15 minutes

Cooking Time: 45 minutes

Serving Time: 60 minutes

Nutritional Info: (Per serving) Calories: 200, Protein: 3g, Fat: 15g, Carbs: 18g

Instructions:

- Preheat the oven to 375°F (190°C).
- Brush the inside of the spaghetti squash with olive oil and season with salt and pepper.
- Roast the squash for 40-45 minutes until tender.

- Scrape the squash with a fork to create spaghetti-like strands.
- Toss with cherry tomatoes and pesto.
- Garnish with fresh basil before serving.

Serving Methods:

1. Sprinkle with pine nuts for added crunch.
2. Serve alongside grilled chicken or fish for a complete meal.

Cucumber and Avocado Gazpacho

Ingredients:

- 2 cucumbers, peeled and diced
- 2 avocados, diced
- 1/2 cup red onion, finely chopped
- 2 cloves garlic, minced
- 4 cups low-sodium vegetable broth
- 1/4 cup lime juice
- 2 tablespoons cilantro, chopped
- Salt and pepper to taste

Preparation Time: 15 minutes

Cooking Time: 0 minutes

Serving Time: 15 minutes

Nutritional Info: (Per serving) Calories: 180, Protein: 3g, Fat: 15g, Carbs: 15g

Instructions:

- In a blender, combine cucumbers, avocados, red onion, garlic, vegetable broth, lime juice, cilantro, salt, and pepper.
- Blend until smooth.
- Chill in the refrigerator for at least 2 hours before serving.

Serving Methods:

1. Top with a dollop of Greek yogurt.
2. Garnish with additional cilantro and diced avocado.

Mushroom and Spinach Stuffed Bell Peppers

Ingredients:

- 4 large bell peppers, halved and seeds removed
- 2 cups mushrooms, chopped
- 2 cups spinach, chopped
- 1 cup quinoa, cooked
- 1 cup low-fat feta cheese, crumbled
- 2 tablespoons olive oil
- 1 teaspoon Italian seasoning

- Salt and pepper to taste

Preparation Time: 20 minutes

Cooking Time: 30 minutes

Serving Time: 50 minutes

Nutritional Info: (Per serving, 1 half) Calories: 200, Protein: 10g, Fat: 8g, Carbs: 25g

Instructions:

- Preheat the oven to 375°F (190°C).
- In a skillet, sauté mushrooms and spinach in olive oil until wilted.
- In a large bowl, combine the cooked quinoa, sautéed mushrooms and spinach, feta cheese, Italian seasoning, salt, and pepper.
- Stuff each bell pepper half with the mixture.
- Bake for 25-30 minutes until peppers are tender.

Serving Methods:

1. Serve with a side of tomato salsa.
2. Drizzle with a balsamic reduction for added flavor.

CHAPTER SIX

DINNER RECIPES

Canned Tomato Basil Sauce with Zucchini Noodles

Ingredients:

- 6 cups fresh tomatoes, peeled and diced
- 2 cloves garlic, minced
- 1/4 cup fresh basil, chopped
- 2 tablespoons olive oil
- Salt and pepper to taste
- Zucchini noodles (for serving)

Preparation Time: 20 minutes

Cooking Time: 30 minutes

Serving Time: 50 minutes

Nutritional Info: (Per serving) Calories: 80, Protein: 2g, Fat: 5g, Carbs: 8g

Instructions:

- In a large pot, sauté garlic in olive oil until fragrant.
- Add diced tomatoes, basil, salt, and pepper. Simmer for 25-30 minutes.
- Use a blender to puree the sauce until smooth.

- Serve over zucchini noodles.

Serving Methods:

1. Top with grated Parmesan cheese.
2. Add grilled chicken or shrimp for extra protein.

Lemon Dill Salmon Packets

Ingredients:

- 4 salmon fillets
- 1 lemon, thinly sliced
- 2 tablespoons fresh dill, chopped
- 2 tablespoons olive oil
- Salt and pepper to taste

Preparation Time: 15 minutes

Cooking Time: 20 minutes

Serving Time: 35 minutes

Nutritional Info: (Per serving) Calories: 250, Protein: 25g, Fat: 15g, Carbs: 2g

Instructions:

- Preheat the oven to 375°F (190°C).
- Place each salmon fillet on a piece of foil.
- Drizzle with olive oil, sprinkle with fresh dill, and season with salt and pepper.

- Top with lemon slices and fold the foil to create packets.
- Bake for 15-20 minutes until salmon is cooked through.

Serving Methods:

1. Serve over a bed of steamed broccoli.
2. Accompany with a side of cauliflower rice.

Canned Pickled Cucumbers and Grilled Chicken Salad

Ingredients:

- 2 cups canned pickled cucumbers
- 2 grilled chicken breasts, sliced
- 4 cups mixed greens
- 1/4 cup feta cheese, crumbled
- 2 tablespoons balsamic vinaigrette

Preparation Time: 15 minutes

Cooking Time: 15 minutes (for grilling chicken)

Serving Time: 30 minutes

Nutritional Info: (Per serving) Calories: 300, Protein: 30g, Fat: 12g, Carbs: 18g

Instructions:

- Assemble mixed greens on a plate.

- Top with grilled chicken, pickled cucumbers, and feta cheese.

- Drizzle with balsamic vinaigrette before serving.

Serving Methods:

1. Add cherry tomatoes for extra color and flavor.
2. Sprinkle with chopped almonds for crunch.

Eggplant and Chickpea Stew

Ingredients:

- 2 medium eggplants, diced
- 1 can (15 oz.) chickpeas, drained and rinsed
- 1 onion, chopped
- 2 cloves garlic, minced
- 2 cans (14 oz. each) diced tomatoes
- 2 tablespoons olive oil
- 1 teaspoon cumin
- Salt and pepper to taste

Preparation Time: 20 minutes

Cooking Time: 30 minutes

Serving Time: 50 minutes

Nutritional Info: (Per serving) Calories: 180, Protein: 5g, Fat: 8g, Carbs: 25g

Instructions:

- In a large pot, sauté onions and garlic in olive oil until softened.
- Add diced eggplant, chickpeas, diced tomatoes, cumin, salt, and pepper.
- Simmer for 25-30 minutes until vegetables are tender.
- Serve hot.

Serving Methods:

1. Top with a dollop of Greek yogurt.
2. Serve over a bed of quinoa or cauliflower rice.

Canned Green Bean Almondine

Ingredients:

- 4 cups canned green beans
- 1/2 cup slivered almonds
- 2 tablespoons olive oil
- 1 tablespoon lemon juice
- Salt and pepper to taste

Preparation Time: 15 minutes

Cooking Time: 10 minutes

Serving Time: 25 minutes

Nutritional Info: (Per serving) Calories: 120, Protein: 4g, Fat: 10g, Carbs: 8g

Instructions:

- In a skillet, toast slivered almonds until golden brown.
- Add canned green beans, olive oil, lemon juice, salt, and pepper.
- Sauté for 5-7 minutes until beans are heated through.
- Serve warm.

Serving Methods:

1. Sprinkle with fresh parsley for added freshness.
2. Top with crumbled feta cheese.

Mushroom and Spinach Quiche with Almond Flour Crust

Ingredients:

- 2 cups mushrooms, sliced
- 2 cups fresh spinach, chopped
- 1 cup almond flour

- 4 eggs
- 1 cup unsweetened almond milk
- 1/2 cup grated Parmesan cheese
- 2 tablespoons olive oil
- Salt and pepper to taste

Preparation Time: 30 minutes

Cooking Time: 40 minutes

Serving Time: 70 minutes

Nutritional Info: (Per serving) Calories: 220, Protein: 12g, Fat: 18g, Carbs: 6g

Instructions:

- Preheat the oven to 375°F (190°C).
- In a skillet, sauté mushrooms and spinach in olive oil until wilted.
- In a bowl, combine almond flour, eggs, almond milk, Parmesan cheese, salt, and pepper.
- Press the mixture into a pie dish to form a crust.
- Spread the mushroom and spinach mixture over the crust.
- Bake for 35-40 minutes until the quiche is set.

Serving Methods:

1. Serve with a side of mixed greens.

2. Top with a dollop of sour cream or Greek yogurt.

Turkey and Vegetable Stir-Fry with Cauliflower Rice

Ingredients:

- 1 lb ground turkey
- 2 cups broccoli florets
- 1 cup bell peppers (any color), sliced
- 1 cup snow peas, trimmed
- 2 tablespoons low-sodium soy sauce
- 1 tablespoon sesame oil
- 1 teaspoon ginger, minced
- 4 cups cauliflower rice (for serving)

Preparation Time: 20 minutes

Cooking Time: 20 minutes

Serving Time: 40 minutes

Nutritional Info: (Per serving) Calories: 250, Protein: 25g, Fat: 10g, Carbs: 15g

Instructions:

- In a skillet, cook ground turkey until browned.

- Add broccoli, bell peppers, snow peas, soy sauce, sesame oil, and ginger. Stir until vegetables are tender.
- Serve the stir-fry over cauliflower rice.

Serving Methods:

1. Garnish with sliced green onions.
2. Sprinkle with sesame seeds for added texture.

Canned Roasted Red Pepper and Artichoke Chicken

Ingredients:

- 4 boneless, skinless chicken breasts
- 1 jar (12 oz.) roasted red peppers, drained and sliced
- 1 can (14 oz.) artichoke hearts, drained and quartered
- 2 tablespoons olive oil
- 2 cloves garlic, minced
- 1 teaspoon dried oregano
- Salt and pepper to taste

Preparation Time: 15 minutes

Cooking Time: 25 minutes

Serving Time: 40 minutes

Nutritional Info: (Per serving) Calories: 280, Protein: 30g, Fat: 12g, Carbs: 10g

Instructions:

- Preheat the oven to 400°F (200°C).
- Season chicken breasts with salt, pepper, and oregano.
- In a skillet, sear chicken in olive oil until browned on both sides.
- Transfer chicken to a baking dish and top with sliced roasted red peppers and quartered artichoke hearts.
- Bake for 20-25 minutes until chicken is cooked through.

Serving Methods:

1. Serve over a bed of sautéed spinach.
2. Accompany with a side of quinoa or brown rice.

Cabbage and Turkey Stuffed Peppers

Ingredients:

- 4 bell peppers, halved and seeds removed
- 1 lb ground turkey
- 2 cups cabbage, shredded

- 1 cup cauliflower rice
- 1 can (14 oz.) diced tomatoes, drained
- 1 teaspoon paprika
- Salt and pepper to taste

Preparation Time: 30 minutes

Cooking Time: 30 minutes

Serving Time: 60 minutes

Nutritional Info: (Per serving, 1 half) Calories: 220, Protein: 25g, Fat: 10g, Carbs: 15g

Instructions:

- Preheat the oven to 375°F (190°C).
- In a skillet, cook ground turkey until browned.
- Add shredded cabbage, cauliflower rice, diced tomatoes, paprika, salt, and pepper. Stir until vegetables are tender.
- Fill each bell pepper half with the turkey and cabbage mixture.
- Bake for 25-30 minutes until peppers are tender.

Serving Methods:

1. Top with a dollop of Greek yogurt.
2. Sprinkle with fresh parsley for added flavor.

Canned Beet and Walnut Salad with Grilled Chicken

Ingredients:

- 2 cups canned beets, sliced
- 1 cup walnuts, chopped
- 4 cups mixed salad greens
- 2 grilled chicken breasts, sliced
- 1/4 cup balsamic vinaigrette

Preparation Time: 15 minutes

Cooking Time: 15 minutes (for grilling chicken)

Serving Time: 30 minutes

Nutritional Info: (Per serving) Calories: 300, Protein: 20g, Fat: 20g, Carbs: 15g

Instructions:

- Assemble mixed salad greens on a plate.
- Top with sliced beets, chopped walnuts, and grilled chicken.
- Drizzle with balsamic vinaigrette before serving.

Serving Methods:

1. Crumble goat cheese on top for added creaminess.

2. Garnish with pomegranate seeds for a burst of
    flavor.

75

CHAPTER SEVEN

SNACK RECIPES

Canned Roasted Red Pepper Hummus

Ingredients:

- 1 can (15 oz.) chickpeas, drained and rinsed
- 1/2 cup roasted red peppers, drained
- 2 tablespoons tahini
- 2 cloves garlic, minced
- 3 tablespoons olive oil
- 2 tablespoons lemon juice
- Salt and pepper to taste
- Carrot and cucumber sticks (for serving)

Preparation Time: 10 minutes

Cooking Time: 0 minutes

Serving Time: 10 minutes

Nutritional Info: (Per serving) Calories: 120, Protein: 4g, Fat: 8g, Carbs: 10g

Instructions:

- In a food processor, blend chickpeas, roasted red peppers, tahini, garlic, olive oil, lemon juice, salt, and pepper until smooth.

- Transfer to a jar for canning.

- Serve with carrot and cucumber sticks.

Serving Methods:

1. Spread on whole-grain crackers.

2. Use as a dip for cherry tomatoes.

Canned Pickled Radishes

Ingredients:

- 2 bunches radishes, thinly sliced

- 1 cup white vinegar

- 1/2 cup water

- 2 tablespoons honey

- 1 teaspoon mustard seeds

- 1 teaspoon salt

- Fresh dill (for garnish)

Preparation Time: 15 minutes

Cooking Time: 5 minutes

Serving Time: 20 minutes

Nutritional Info: (Per serving) Calories: 20, Protein: 0g, Fat: 0g, Carbs: 5g

Instructions:

- In a saucepan, combine vinegar, water, honey, mustard seeds, and salt. Bring to a boil.
- Add sliced radishes and simmer for 3-5 minutes.
- Pack the pickled radishes into jars for canning, topping with fresh dill.
- Allow to cool before serving.

Serving Methods:

1. Serve as a tangy side to cheese and crackers.
2. Top avocado toast with pickled radishes.

Spiced Pumpkin Seed Snack

Ingredients:

- 2 cups pumpkin seeds (pepitas), cleaned
- 1 tablespoon olive oil
- 1 teaspoon cumin
- 1 teaspoon paprika
- 1/2 teaspoon cayenne pepper
- Salt to taste

Preparation Time: 10 minutes

Cooking Time: 10 minutes

Serving Time: 20 minutes

Nutritional Info: (Per serving) Calories: 180, Protein: 10g, Fat: 15g, Carbs: 5g

Instructions:

- Preheat the oven to 350°F (175°C).
- Toss pumpkin seeds with olive oil, cumin, paprika, cayenne pepper, and salt.
- Spread the seeds on a baking sheet and bake for 10 minutes or until golden.
- Allow to cool before storing in jars for canning.

Serving Methods:

1. Sprinkle on top of a mixed green salad.
2. Enjoy as a crunchy topping for yogurt.

Cucumber and Greek Yogurt Dip

Ingredients:

- 2 medium cucumbers, grated and drained
- 1 cup Greek yogurt
- 2 cloves garlic, minced
- 2 tablespoons fresh dill, chopped
- 1 tablespoon lemon juice
- Salt and pepper to taste

- Whole grain pita wedges (for serving)

Preparation Time: 15 minutes

Cooking Time: 0 minutes

Serving Time: 15 minutes

Nutritional Info: (Per serving) Calories: 80, Protein: 5g, Fat: 2g, Carbs: 10g

Instructions:

- In a bowl, combine grated and drained cucumbers, Greek yogurt, garlic, dill, lemon juice, salt, and pepper.
- Transfer to jars for canning.
- Serve with whole grain pita wedges.

Serving Methods:

1. Spread on cucumber slices for a low-carb option.
2. Use as a refreshing dressing for a chopped salad.

Canned Roasted Chickpeas

Ingredients:

- 2 cans (15 oz. each) chickpeas, drained and rinsed
- 2 tablespoons olive oil
- 1 teaspoon cumin

- 1 teaspoon paprika

- 1/2 teaspoon garlic powder

- Salt to taste

Preparation Time: 10 minutes

Cooking Time: 30 minutes

Serving Time: 40 minutes

Nutritional Info: (Per serving) Calories: 120, Protein: 5g, Fat: 5g, Carbs: 15g

Instructions:

- Preheat the oven to 400°F (200°C).

- Toss chickpeas with olive oil, cumin, paprika, garlic powder, and salt.

- Spread on a baking sheet and roast for 25-30 minutes until crispy.

- Allow to cool before storing in jars for canning.

Serving Methods:

1. Sprinkle over a green salad.
2. Enjoy as a protein-packed snack on its own.

Canned Roasted Garlic and Rosemary Almonds

Ingredients:

- 2 cups raw almonds
- 2 tablespoons olive oil
- 3 cloves garlic, minced
- 1 tablespoon fresh rosemary, chopped
- Salt to taste

Preparation Time: 10 minutes

Cooking Time: 15 minutes

Serving Time: 25 minutes

Nutritional Info: (Per serving) Calories: 200, Protein: 7g, Fat: 17g, Carbs: 7g

Instructions:

- Preheat the oven to 350°F (175°C).
- Toss almonds with olive oil, minced garlic, rosemary, and salt.
- Spread on a baking sheet and roast for 12-15 minutes until golden.
- Allow to cool before storing in jars for canning.

Serving Methods:

1. Pair with a variety of cheeses for a charcuterie board.
2. Add to a trail mix with dried fruits.

Canned Zucchini Chips

Ingredients:

- 2 medium zucchinis, thinly sliced
- 2 tablespoons olive oil
- 1 teaspoon garlic powder
- 1 teaspoon onion powder
- 1/2 teaspoon paprika
- Salt to taste

Preparation Time: 15 minutes

Cooking Time: 2 hours (oven or dehydrator)

Serving Time: 2 hours and 15 minutes

Nutritional Info: (Per serving) Calories: 80, Protein: 2g, Fat: 7g, Carbs: 5g

Instructions:

- Preheat the oven to 200°F (95°C) or set a dehydrator to 135°F (57°C).
- Toss zucchini slices with olive oil, garlic powder, onion powder, paprika, and salt.
- Arrange on a baking sheet or dehydrator tray.
- Bake or dehydrate for 2 hours until crispy.
- Allow to cool before storing in jars for canning.

Serving Methods:

1. Dip in the cucumber and Greek yogurt dip.

2. Enjoy as a guilt-free alternative to potato chips.

Canned Mango Salsa

Ingredients:

- 2 ripe mangoes, diced

- 1/2 cup red onion, finely chopped

- 1 jalapeño, seeded and minced

- 1/4 cup fresh cilantro, chopped

- Juice of 2 limes

- Salt to taste

- Baked whole grain tortilla chips (for serving)

Preparation Time: 15 minutes

Cooking Time: 0 minutes

Serving Time: 15 minutes

Nutritional Info: (Per serving) Calories: 60, Protein: 1g, Fat: 0g, Carbs: 15g

Instructions:

- In a bowl, combine diced mangoes, red onion, jalapeño, cilantro, lime juice, and salt.

- Transfer to jars for canning.

- Serve with baked whole grain tortilla chips.

Serving Methods:

1. Top grilled chicken or fish with mango salsa.
2. Use as a refreshing topping for tacos.

Canned Cinnamon Apple Chips

Ingredients:

- 4 apples, thinly sliced
- 1 tablespoon lemon juice
- 1 teaspoon ground cinnamon
- 1/2 teaspoon nutmeg
- 1 tablespoon honey (optional)
- Baked whole grain pita chips (for serving)

Preparation Time: 15 minutes

Cooking Time: 2 hours (oven or dehydrator)

Serving Time: 2 hours and 15 minutes

Nutritional Info: (Per serving) Calories: 80, Protein: 1g, Fat: 0g, Carbs: 20g

Instructions:

- Preheat the oven to 200°F (95°C) or set a dehydrator to 135°F (57°C).

- Toss apple slices with lemon juice, cinnamon, nutmeg, and honey (if using).
- Arrange on a baking sheet or dehydrator tray.
- Bake or dehydrate for 2 hours until crispy.
- Allow to cool before storing in jars for canning.

Serving Methods:

1. Sprinkle over oatmeal or yogurt.
2. Enjoy as a sweet and crunchy standalone snack.

Canned Beet and Goat Cheese Dip

Ingredients:

- 1 can (15 oz.) beets, drained
- 4 oz. goat cheese
- 1/4 cup walnuts, chopped
- 1 tablespoon balsamic vinegar
- Salt and pepper to taste
- Whole grain crackers (for serving)

Preparation Time: 10 minutes

Cooking Time: 0 minutes

Serving Time: 10 minutes

Nutritional Info: (Per serving) Calories: 120, Protein: 4g, Fat: 8g, Carbs: 8g

Instructions:

- In a food processor, blend drained beets, goat cheese, chopped walnuts, balsamic vinegar, salt, and pepper until smooth.
- Transfer to jars for canning.
- Serve with whole grain crackers.

Serving Methods:

1. Spread on sliced cucumber rounds.
2. Use as a unique spread for sandwiches or wraps.

CHAPTER EIGHT
MEAL PLAN

Day 1:

Breakfast: Vegetable Omelette with Canned Tomato Basil Sauce

Lunch: Turkey and Vegetable Lettuce Wraps

Dinner: Canned Roasted Red Pepper and Artichoke Chicken

Snack: Canned Roasted Chickpeas

Day 2:

Breakfast: Spaghetti Squash with Pesto and Cherry Tomatoes

Lunch: Salmon and Asparagus Foil Packets

Dinner: Canned Zucchini Chips with Cucumber and Greek Yogurt Dip

Snack: Spiced Pumpkin Seed Snack

Day 3:

Breakfast: Cauliflower and Broccoli Soup

Lunch: Mushroom and Spinach Stuffed Bell Peppers

Dinner: Canned Pickled Cucumbers and Grilled Chicken Salad

Snack: Canned Mango Salsa with Baked Whole Grain Tortilla Chips

Day 4:

Breakfast: Eggplant and Chickpea Stew

Lunch: Turkey and Vegetable Stir-Fry with Cauliflower Rice

Dinner: Canned Cinnamon Apple Chips with Beet and Goat Cheese Dip

Snack: Canned Roasted Garlic and Rosemary Almonds

Day 5:

Breakfast: Lemon Dill Salmon Packets

Lunch: Cabbage and Turkey Stuffed Peppers

Dinner: Canned Pickled Radishes with Canned Beet and Walnut Salad

Snack: Canned Beet and Goat Cheese Dip with Whole Grain Crackers

Day 6:

Breakfast: Mushroom and Spinach Quiche with Almond Flour Crust

Lunch: Canned Green Bean Almondine

Dinner: Canned Tomato Basil Sauce with Zucchini Noodles

Snack: Canned Spiced Pumpkin Seed Snack

Day 7:

Breakfast: Cucumber and Avocado Gazpacho

Lunch: Canned Roasted Chickpeas with Greek Salad

Dinner: Canned Roasted Red Pepper Hummus with Crudites

Snack: Canned Cinnamon Apple Chips

Day 8:

Breakfast: Canned Pickled Radishes with Scrambled Eggs

Lunch: Spaghetti Squash with Pesto and Cherry Tomatoes

Dinner: Canned Zucchini Chips with Cucumber and Greek Yogurt Dip

Snack: Canned Spiced Pumpkin Seed Snack

Day 9:

Breakfast: Eggplant and Chickpea Stew

Lunch: Turkey and Vegetable Stir-Fry with Cauliflower Rice

Dinner: Canned Cinnamon Apple Chips with Beet and Goat Cheese Dip

Snack: Canned Beet and Goat Cheese Dip with Whole Grain Crackers

Day 10:

Breakfast: Salmon and Asparagus Foil Packets

Lunch: Cabbage and Turkey Stuffed Peppers

Dinner: Canned Pickled Cucumbers and Grilled Chicken Salad

Snack: Canned Mango Salsa with Baked Whole Grain Tortilla Chips

Day 11:

Breakfast: Lemon Dill Salmon Packets

Lunch: Mushroom and Spinach Stuffed Bell Peppers

Dinner: Canned Roasted Red Pepper and Artichoke Chicken

Snack: Canned Roasted Chickpeas

Day 12:

Breakfast: Cauliflower and Broccoli Soup

Lunch: Turkey and Vegetable Lettuce Wraps

Dinner: Canned Zucchini Chips with Cucumber and Greek Yogurt Dip

Snack: Spiced Pumpkin Seed Snack

Day 13:

Breakfast: Vegetable Omelette with Canned Tomato Basil Sauce

Lunch: Canned Roasted Chickpeas with Greek Salad

Dinner: Canned Roasted Red Pepper Hummus with Crudites

Snack: Canned Cinnamon Apple Chips

Day 14:

Breakfast: Cucumber and Avocado Gazpacho

Lunch: Spaghetti Squash with Pesto and Cherry Tomatoes

Dinner: Canned Pickled Radishes with Canned Beet and Walnut Salad

Snack: Canned Pickled Cucumbers and Grilled Chicken Salad

Day 15:

Breakfast: Mushroom and Spinach Quiche with Almond Flour Crust

Lunch: Canned Green Bean Almondine

Dinner: Canned Tomato Basil Sauce with Zucchini Noodles

Snack: Canned Mango Salsa with Baked Whole Grain Tortilla Chips

Day 16:

Breakfast: Canned Pickled Radishes with Scrambled Eggs

Lunch: Turkey and Vegetable Stir-Fry with Cauliflower Rice

Dinner: Canned Beet and Goat Cheese Dip with Whole Grain Crackers

Snack: Canned Spiced Pumpkin Seed Snack

Day 17:

Breakfast: Eggplant and Chickpea Stew

Lunch: Cabbage and Turkey Stuffed Peppers

Dinner: Canned Cinnamon Apple Chips with Beet and Goat Cheese Dip

Snack: Canned Roasted Garlic and Rosemary Almonds

Day 18:

Breakfast: Salmon and Asparagus Foil Packets

Lunch: Canned Roasted Chickpeas with Greek Salad

Dinner: Canned Roasted Red Pepper Hummus with Crudites

Snack: Canned Mango Salsa with Baked Whole Grain Tortilla Chips

Day 19:

Breakfast: Cauliflower and Broccoli Soup

Lunch: Turkey and Vegetable Lettuce Wraps

Dinner: Canned Zucchini Chips with Cucumber and Greek Yogurt Dip

Snack: Spiced Pumpkin Seed Snack

Day 20:

Breakfast: Vegetable Omelette with Canned Tomato Basil Sauce

Lunch: Canned Roasted Chickpeas with Greek Salad

Dinner: Canned Tomato Basil Sauce with Zucchini Noodles

Snack: Canned Pickled Cucumbers and Grilled Chicken Salad

Day 21:

Breakfast: Mushroom and Spinach Quiche with Almond Flour Crust

Lunch: Canned Pickled Radishes with Canned Beet and Walnut Salad

Dinner: Canned Roasted Red Pepper and Artichoke Chicken

Snack: Canned Beet and Goat Cheese Dip with Whole Grain Crackers

CHAPTER NINE

TIPS FOR SUCCESS ON A LOW OXALATE DIET

Reading Food Labels

Navigating food labels becomes even more crucial when following a low oxalate diet. Let's explore a guide to reading food labels for success on a low oxalate diet, with a character named Emily:

Meet Emily, a health-conscious individual committed to maintaining a low oxalate diet for her well-being. Armed with the knowledge that oxalates can impact kidney health, Emily approaches food labels with a keen eye and a determination to make informed choices.

- **Oxalate Content:**

Emily starts by checking the oxalate content on the label. While not all labels explicitly list oxalate levels, she looks for keywords like "oxalate" or ingredients high in oxalates, such as spinach, beets, or nuts.

- **Serving Size Awareness:**

Emily pays attention to the serving size, ensuring it aligns with her dietary goals. Adjusting portion sizes based on the oxalate content per serving helps her manage her daily oxalate intake effectively.

- **Calcium and Oxalate Ratio:**

Emily considers the calcium and oxalate ratio in foods. Consuming calcium-rich foods alongside moderate oxalate foods can help bind oxalates in the digestive tract, reducing their absorption.

- **Limiting High Oxalate Ingredients:**

Emily scans the ingredient list for high oxalate foods, such as spinach, rhubarb, or almonds. Being vigilant about these ingredients allows her to avoid unexpected sources of oxalates.

- **Awareness of Hidden Oxalates:**

Emily is aware that certain food additives or preservatives may contain hidden oxalates. She reads labels carefully to spot additives like sodium or potassium oxalate, making conscious choices to limit their intake.

- **Calcium Additives:**

Emily looks out for calcium-containing additives or fortifications. While calcium can be beneficial for managing oxalates, it's important to be mindful of the total calcium intake from all sources.

- Low-Oxalate Alternatives:

Emily explores low-oxalate alternatives to high-oxalate foods. For example, she chooses rice over high-oxalate grains or opts for low-oxalate vegetables like kale or broccoli.

- **Limiting Processed and Packaged Foods:**

Emily understands that processed and packaged foods may contain hidden sources of oxalates. She leans towards whole, unprocessed foods to have better control over her oxalate intake.

- **Variety and Nutrient Density:**

Emily ensures a variety of nutrient-dense foods in her low oxalate diet. She selects a wide range of fruits, vegetables, and grains to maintain a balanced and wholesome nutritional profile.

- **Monitoring Sodium and Sugar:**

Emily keeps an eye on sodium and sugar content. While not directly.

Dining Out Strategies

Dining out while adhering to a low oxalate diet requires a strategic approach to make choices that align with your dietary goals. Let's explore some dining-out strategies for success on a low oxalate diet, with a character named James:

Meet James, a health-conscious individual who is committed to maintaining a low oxalate diet even when dining out. James understands that making informed choices at restaurants is essential for keeping his oxalate intake in check and ensuring a positive dining experience.

- **Research Restaurants in Advance:**

James takes the time to research restaurants in advance. Many establishments now provide their menu online, allowing him to review options and choose a restaurant that offers low oxalate choices.

- **Communicate with the Server:**

James communicates with the server about his dietary preferences. He politely asks about the preparation methods, ingredient substitutions, and whether the chef can accommodate a low oxalate request.

- **Choose Calcium-Rich Options:**

James opts for calcium-rich options on the menu. Foods high in calcium can help bind oxalates in the digestive tract, reducing their absorption. He may choose dishes with dairy or other calcium-containing ingredients.

- **Customize Your Order:**

James feels comfortable customizing his order to meet his low oxalate needs. Whether it's asking for specific vegetables or requesting the exclusion of high-oxalate ingredients, he knows that many restaurants are willing to accommodate.

- **Favor Grilled or Steamed Options:**

James leans towards grilled or steamed options. These cooking methods are often associated with fewer added ingredients and less likelihood of high-oxalate components.

- **Be Mindful of Sauces and Dressings:**

James is cautious about sauces and dressings, as they can sometimes contain high-oxalate ingredients. He may request dressings on the side or inquire about alternatives with lower oxalate content.

- **Opt for Low-Oxalate Sides:**

James pays attention to side dishes. Choosing low-oxalate sides, such as baked potatoes instead of spinach, allows him to enjoy a well-rounded meal while managing his oxalate intake.

- **Enjoy Protein-Based Options:**

James often gravitates towards protein-based options. Whether it's lean meats, fish, or poultry, these choices provide essential nutrients without the concern of high oxalate content.

- **Ask for Nutritional Information:**

James is not afraid to ask for nutritional information. Some restaurants provide detailed information about their menu items, helping him make more informed choices based on oxalate content.

- **Bring a Low-Oxalate Snack:**

James may bring a low-oxalate snack, especially if he anticipates limited options on the menu. This ensures he can enjoy a satisfying meal without compromising his dietary goals.

- **Stay Hydrated:**

James stays hydrated by choosing water or other low-oxalate beverages. Hydration is essential for overall health and can support kidney function.

- **Enjoy the Dining Experience:**

Lastly, James focuses on enjoying the dining experience. By planning ahead, communicating effectively, and making thoughtful choices, he can savor the flavors of a delicious meal while maintaining his low oxalate lifestyle.

Managing Cravings and Temptations

Managing cravings and resisting temptations can be challenging, especially when following a low oxalate diet. Let's explore some strategies for success in handling cravings and staying on track, with a character named Olivia:

Meet Olivia, a determined individual committed to maintaining a low oxalate diet for her health. Olivia understands that managing cravings is a crucial aspect of staying consistent with her dietary goals.

- **Understand Cravings:**

Olivia takes the time to understand her cravings. Whether they stem from emotional triggers, habits, or physiological needs, acknowledging and understanding the source of cravings is the first step.

- **Plan Balanced Meals:**

Olivia plans balanced meals that include a variety of nutrient-dense, low oxalate foods. A well-rounded and satisfying diet can help reduce overall cravings and keep her feeling satiated.

- **Stay Hydrated:**

Olivia prioritizes hydration. Sometimes, feelings of hunger can be mistaken for dehydration. Drinking water throughout the day helps curb unnecessary cravings.

- **Incorporate Low-Oxalate Treats:**

Olivia finds or creates low oxalate treat alternatives for her favorite indulgences. Whether it's a low oxalate dessert recipe or a snack, having satisfying alternatives can help manage cravings.

- **Practice Mindful Eating:**

Olivia practices mindful eating. Taking the time to savor each bite, appreciating flavors and textures, can enhance the eating experience and reduce the desire for excessive or unhealthy foods.

- **Distract Yourself:**

When cravings strike, Olivia finds ways to distract herself. Engaging in activities she enjoys, such as reading, taking a walk, or pursuing a hobby, can redirect her focus away from cravings.

- **Keep Low-Oxalate Snacks Handy:**

Olivia keeps low oxalate snacks readily available. Having healthy options on hand makes it easier to resist the temptation of high-oxalate or less desirable choices.

- **Set Realistic Goals:**

Olivia sets realistic and achievable goals. Breaking down larger goals into smaller, manageable steps can make the process more attainable, reducing the likelihood of feeling overwhelmed and succumbing to cravings.

- **Practice Portion Control:**

Olivia practices portion control, especially when it comes to treats or higher oxalate foods. Enjoying small portions in moderation allows her to satisfy cravings without compromising her overall dietary goals.

- **Establish a Support System:**

Olivia surrounds herself with a supportive network. Sharing her low oxalate journey with friends, family, or an online community provides encouragement and understanding when faced with challenging cravings.

- **Celebrate Non-Food Rewards:**

Instead of using food as a reward, Olivia celebrates achievements with non-food rewards. This could be a relaxing bath, a favorite activity, or anything else that brings joy without compromising her low oxalate commitment.

- **Forgive Yourself:**

Lastly, Olivia practices self-compassion. If she occasionally gives in to a craving, she forgives herself and focuses on moving forward with her low oxalate lifestyle. One indulgence doesn't define her journey.

CHAPTER TEN

COMBINING EXERCISE WITH A LOW OXALATE DIET FOR WEIGHT LOSS

Types of Exercise to Consider

- **Cardiovascular Exercise:**

Activities: Running, brisk walking, cycling, swimming, or aerobics.

Benefits: Cardiovascular exercises elevate heart rate and burn calories, supporting weight loss. They also enhance overall cardiovascular health.

- **Strength Training:**

Activities: Weightlifting, resistance training, bodyweight exercises (e.g., squats, lunges, push-ups).

Benefits: Strength training builds lean muscle mass, which can increase metabolism and contribute to weight loss. It also helps with overall strength and toning.

- **High-Intensity Interval Training (HIIT):**

Activities: Short bursts of intense exercise followed by brief rest periods.

Benefits: HIIT is effective for calorie burning, fat loss, and improving cardiovascular fitness. It can be a time-efficient option for weight loss.

- **Yoga:**

Activities: Hatha, Vinyasa, or Power Yoga.

Benefits: Yoga promotes flexibility, balance, and mindfulness. It can be a valuable addition to weight loss efforts by reducing stress and supporting mental well-being.

- **Pilates:**

Activities: Mat exercises or using specialized equipment.

Benefits: Pilates focuses on core strength, flexibility, and overall body toning. It complements a low oxalate diet by promoting a balanced and functional physique.

- **Circuit Training:**

Activities: A combination of strength and aerobic exercises performed consecutively.

Benefits: Circuit training offers a full-body workout, combining the benefits of strength and cardiovascular exercises. It can enhance calorie burning and muscle toning.

Dance Workouts:

Activities: Zumba, dance aerobics, or dance-based fitness classes.

Benefits: Dance workouts make exercise enjoyable while providing cardiovascular benefits. They can be a fun way to burn calories and support weight loss.

- **Walking or Hiking:**

Activities: Brisk walking or hiking in nature.

Benefits: Walking is a low-impact exercise that aids in weight management. Hiking provides additional benefits of being outdoors and engaging various muscle groups.

- **Swimming:**

Activities: Swimming laps or water aerobics.

Benefits: Swimming is a full-body workout that is gentle on the joints. It supports weight loss by burning calories and improving cardiovascular health.

Importance of Physical Activity for Weight Management

Physical activity plays a crucial role in weight management and overall well-being. Let's explore the importance of incorporating regular exercise into a weight management plan:

- **Calorie Expenditure:**

Explanation: Physical activity helps burn calories, contributing to a negative energy balance that is essential for weight loss. It increases the total amount of energy expended by the body, making it easier to create a calorie deficit.

- **Metabolism Boost:**

Explanation: Regular exercise, especially strength training, can boost metabolism by increasing lean muscle mass. A higher metabolism means the body continues to burn calories at an elevated rate even at rest, supporting weight management.

- **Fat Loss vs. Muscle Preservation:**

Explanation: Exercise, particularly resistance training, helps preserve lean muscle mass during weight loss. This is crucial because maintaining muscle mass supports a higher metabolism and contributes to a more toned and healthy physique.

- **Appetite Regulation:**

Explanation: Physical activity can influence appetite hormones, helping regulate hunger and satiety. Regular exercise may reduce cravings and improve the body's ability to respond to internal hunger cues, facilitating better portion control.

- **Improvement in Insulin Sensitivity:**

Explanation: Exercise enhances insulin sensitivity, allowing the body to use glucose more effectively. Improved insulin sensitivity is associated with better blood sugar control and reduced risk of developing type 2 diabetes, which is often linked to obesity.

- **Stress Reduction:**

Explanation: Exercise is a powerful stress-reducer. High stress levels can contribute to overeating or making unhealthy food choices. Engaging in physical activity helps manage stress, promoting a healthier relationship with food and aiding in weight management.

- **Enhanced Cardiovascular Health:**

Explanation: Regular cardiovascular exercise improves heart health and circulation. It reduces the risk of cardiovascular diseases associated with obesity, such as hypertension and heart disease.

- **Promotion of Long-Term Weight Maintenance:**

Explanation: Incorporating exercise into a weight loss plan increases the likelihood of maintaining weight loss over the long term. Sustainable weight management is about adopting a healthy lifestyle that includes regular physical activity.

- **Mood and Mental Well-Being:**

Explanation: Exercise releases endorphins, the body's natural mood lifters. It can alleviate feelings of depression and anxiety, providing mental and emotional benefits that contribute to overall well-being and weight management

CONCLUSION

In conclusion, achieving and maintaining a healthy lifestyle requires a holistic and adaptable approach that encompasses both dietary and exercise considerations. The journey towards optimal health involves understanding the intricate interplay between factors such as nutrition, physical activity, mental well-being, and overall lifestyle choices. Through thoughtful assessment and strategic adjustments, individuals can navigate the path towards their health and fitness goals with greater success.

In the realm of diet, a low oxalate approach, especially when coupled with weight loss objectives, holds potential benefits. Understanding the role of oxalates in the body, evaluating the impact on weight management, and exploring the benefits of a low oxalate diet shed light on a nuanced approach to dietary choices. It's crucial to appreciate the potential advantages, such as reduced inflammation, improved digestion, and enhanced nutrient absorption, while being mindful of the need for a balanced and varied diet to ensure overall well-being.

When it comes to exercise, incorporating a diverse range of activities is key. From cardiovascular exercises to strength training, flexibility work, and mind-body practices, the goal is to create a well-rounded fitness routine. Regular assessments of your exercise routine, considering factors like frequency, intensity, and variety, allow for necessary adjustments to align with your evolving fitness goals and personal preferences.

Beyond the specifics of diet and exercise, monitoring weight loss, assessing energy levels, and evaluating overall well-being provide valuable insights into the effectiveness of your health journey. Regular self-assessment, tracking progress through various indicators, and remaining adaptable to individual needs contribute to a sustainable and balanced approach to health.

Ultimately, the journey towards optimal health is dynamic and unique to each individual. It involves a commitment to continuous learning, self-awareness, and the willingness to make adjustments as needed. Whether you're managing weight, improving energy levels, or enhancing overall well-being, the key is to embrace a comprehensive and personalized approach that integrates mindful dietary choices, regular physical activity, and a commitment to long-term health and vitality.